Fasting Diet

For Weight Loss

By Dwayne Whiting

Table Of Contents

Introduction

I want to thank you and congratulate you for downloading the book, "Fasting Diet for Weight Loss".

This book would provide you with information on how you can use fasting as a means to losing weight but without having to risk your own health. Contrary to what some may believe, fasting can be done properly and this would help you avoid potential health problems.

Fasting has gained quite the notorious reputation for being a dangerous form of dieting but how true is this? You'll be surprised to know that it isn't as risky as some people make it seem, as long as you do it in moderation and remember certain things-- you'll be just fine and the best bit? You will lose weight.

Thanks again for downloading this book, I hope you enjoy it!

Chapter 1: An Introduction

Fasting, as you may or may not know, is actually an age-old practice for many, though it is often done for religious reasons. When it comes to weight loss, however, it still manages to capture the attention of many as one of the quickest, and most efficient ways of losing weight within a short period of time. But the question remains, is it safe? The truth is simple, depending on how a person approaches fasting for weight loss, it can go both ways. A quick search online would show you just how widely debated this is.

Here's another fact, fasting can be done properly and safely, and you will lose weight through it. There are many different ways through which this can be done and many diet plans have also incorporated it into their programs. From detoxifying and flushing toxins out of the body by not eating solids to simply not eating for a few hours each day, this can all be considered as a form of fasting. But what's the basic idea for it?

Fasting means eating little to no food at all for a few days or in some cases, a few hours. It is recommended that you don't do the zero food kind of fasting especially if you do a lot within a day. Your body will need some for of sustenance, after all, and you can't simply disregard your daily nutritional needs. What you need is a fasting plan that would allow you to receive these nutrients but would also ensure that you burn more calories than you eat. Remember, not all fasting diets are created equal, there is a safe way of doing this.

First off, who should avoid it? Fasting isn't recommended for the elderly, any individual who have a chronic disease as well as women who are currently pregnant. This is certainly a no-no for diabetics. As for healthy adults, it is unlikely to be dangerous.

Now, fasting for a few days wouldn't hurt you if you're healthy and make sure that you keep yourself hydrated. 3 to 4 days would still be good but anything longer can be quite bad for you. Why? As we have pointed out earlier, your body requires vitamins and minerals along with other nutrients in order to function properly and stay healthy. Should you not get them, you might experience certain symptoms such as dizziness, dehydration, fatigue and constipation. You may also lose some of your ability to tolerate colder weather.

Another important thing that you must remember, before you get started with fasting is to talk to your doctor about it. He or she would be able to provide you with an assessment and advise you on whether or not this is good for you. Once you've been given the go-signal, you can then get started with fasting diet plan. A plan is important, of course, as you wouldn't want to do things blindly and fumble about. What are some of the things that you need to keep in mind when it comes to creating a diet plan? Well, if you're not going to work with a dietitian, keep these things in mind:

1. Work out how many days you will be fasting.

2. Think about the kind of of work that you will be participating in during those days. It is recommended that you do very light work while fasting as doing too much, considering the lack of fuel in your body, can lead to dizziness and fatigue.

3. Make sure that you include proper hydration as well as supplements where you'll be getting energy from.

Light snacks at least twice a day would be helpful and would not harm your weight loss goals whatsoever.

Now that you have the basics down, let's talk more about how fasting can be beneficial to your weight loss goals as well as overall health if you do it properly.

Chapter 2: The Benefits

Rare are the times that you will find fasting and health benefits in the same sentence. The reason for this is simple, many people believe it to be an unhealthy way of losing weight. However, this book would help you understand that this is not the case at all. One simply needs to remember moderation and fasting properly, without having to risk one's health.

Let's talk about what short fasting can do. Fasting for a few days can, in fact, reduce your oxidative stress as well as lessen any inflammation in your cells. Professionals have theorized that this can actually help in preventing as well as repairing any DNA damage which could eventually turn into cancer if left untreated. There are also studies that suggest fasting to be another way of slowing down our body's internal clock. In other words, it helps delay aging. Not merely skin-wise, it can also keep our internal organs youthful and functioning efficiently.

Quite interesting, right? Well, the benefits don't stop there.

1. Fasting helps promote detoxification. The processed food we eat every single day contains a number of different additives and these, eventually turn into toxins which damage our body. Some of them can actually hasten the production of AGE or advanced glycation end products, many of which are stored in our fats. During fasting, fat is burned and these toxins are released and then purged from our body. The kidneys and liver benefit greatly from this detoxification.

2. Fasting allows our digestive system to rest. Whenever we go through fasting, it allows our digestive organs to take a break from breaking down the food that we eat which can be quite tasking. While the physiologic functions still continue, such as the production of various digestive secretions only at greatly reduced rates. How does this benefit us? Well, it allows the body to maintain a proper balance of fluids and the release of energy also begins to follow a gradual pattern. However, fasting does not prevent the production of stomach acids and as such, patients who have been diagnosed with peptic ulcer are advised to avoid fasting.

3. Fasting helps resolve inflammatory response. There have been studies that show how fasting can also promote the resolution of different allergies and inflammatory diseases. A good example of which would be psoriasis and rheumatoid arthritis. There have also been studies that show how it can help when it comes to the healing of inflammatory bowel diseases which include ulcerative colitis.

4. Fasting reduces blood sugar. Fasting is actually capable of increasing the body's breakdown of glucose so that it generates more fuel for energy. At the same time, however, it also reduces its production of insulin this effectively resting the pancreas. In this case, glucagon is produced in order to accommodate the breakdown of glucose thus lowering the levels of blood sugar in our system.

5. Fasting increases fat breakdown. When we fast, the body responds by breaking down glucose, as we have pointed out earlier. However, when the store of

glucose is depleted, ketosis is put into action. This is basically the body's way of breaking down fats in order to use it as fuel for energy. The fats stored in our muscles and in the kidney are the first to be broken down.

6. Fasting corrects high blood pressure. If you're looking for a way to lower your blood pressure without having to resort to taking drugs then fasting is the way to go. It can help in reducing the risk of atherosclerosis or the clogging of our arteries by different fat particles. Whenever we fast, our metabolic rate is also reduced and so the body's fear and flight responses such as adrenaline are also lowered. This helps keep our metabolism steady and right within the limits. The benefit? A reduction in our blood pressure.

7. Fasting promotes efficient weight loss. As we have pointed out and is also the very core of this book, fasting is an efficient method for weight loss. Only if done in moderation, however. If not, this can be quite risky.

8. Fasting promotes a healthier diet and lifestyle. Our body automatically craves for the food that we eat the most and unfortunately, this means processed food for the great majority of us. Now, one would think that fasting would actually increase that craving further but this not whole true. In fact, it has been observed that fasting can help in decreasing our craving for processed foods. This should allow us to put forth the dietary changes that we want, perhaps a switch to something healthier and natural? This can pave the way towards a healthier lifestyle as well.

9. Fasting improves our immunity. You thought only bad things could ever happen when you fast, right? Well, that's not true as well. If you maintain a well-balanced diet in between your fasts, this can actually help improve your immunity. This happens because of the toxins and poisons that are eliminated from your body thus allowing it to function better. The same can be said whenever fat stores get exhausted, not only will you feel lighter, you will also have more energy. So, if you choose to eat a fruit as a means of breaking your fast, you're actually increasing your body's storage of vitamins and minerals which then improves your immunity.

10. Fasting can help an individual overcome certain addictions. Yes, you read that right. Fasting has been found to be quite helpful when it comes to reducing cravings for different things such as caffeine, alcohol, nicotine as well as other addictive substances. Whilst other regimens would be needed to completely resolve these things, fasting can still play a big part when it comes to getting there. At the same time, you're also detoxifying and healing your body of the damages that your habit has done to it. That's hitting two birds with one stone! You need not fast for too long, however, you can take breaks. But doing it with regularity can train your system to not crave for these things anymore.

Chapter 3: Types of Fasting

When it comes to the actual fasting, there are many different kinds but they all offer the same benefits of detoxification and healing. However, since people have different preferences as well, this variety enables them to pick and choose which one fits them the best. There is no such thing as the best when it comes to fasting, it all depends upon the person's needs and lifestyle. After all, it has to fit or they might have some trouble adjusting to it.

Fasting Methods 101:

1. Dry Fasting – This is also known as the Black Fast, the Hebrew Fast and the Absolute fast. It is one of the more extreme varieties and finds its roots in something more spiritual where one needs to forego eating food or drinking water for a period of time. This, ladies and gents, is something that you shouldn't try just to lose some weight. People do this as an act of penance and for good reason, it is torturous to the body and could lead to a number of complications. So, remember, never do a dry fast.

2. Liquid Fasting – As the name itself implies, this fast involves liquids only. There are two different kinds. The first of which, would be water fasting and it is also one of the oldest forms of liquid fasting. It is of great therapeutic benefit and detoxifies the body in a short span of time. However, for beginners, this can be quite difficult to commit to since we all appreciate a little texture in what we eat. Juice fasting is another popular form of liquid fasting and is also prevalent in Hollywood with stars such as Kim Kardashian and

Beyonce using it to help them drop the baby weight that they have gained. Fruits and vegetables used in this provide the body with the necessary nutrients it needs. The Master Cleanse or the Lemonade Diet is one of the newer approaches and is also one of the most popular.

3. Partial Fasting – Also often referred to as a selective fast, this type of fasting would have you eat some solid food. It's not the amount that matters, but he kind. In this case, certain food types would be limited or completely excluded from your daily diet. Cleansing diets as well as mono-diets such as rice fasting are considered to be partial fasts.

Juice and fruit fasts tend to be more gentle to the body as the detoxification happens more gradually. The side effects aren't very extreme and the most you'll feel is a slight headache. However, this varies depending on your current health condition. Weigh the options and take a good look at your currently lifestyle, and how much you're willing to sacrifice for the period you'll be fasting.

Fasting will inevitably bring forth certain cleansing and detoxification symptoms which might get in the way of your daily activities. You might have less energy than before and so on. This is something that you'll need to discuss with your physician as well to make sure that you're well aware of the possible consequences and to ascertain that your body can handle it.

One of the best ways through which you can get this started is through fruit or juice fasts. You can do this at least once a week until the symptoms begin to lessen. From there, you can also try something more advance though this isn't necessarily the next step that you should take. Continuing with the lighter fasts should serve you just as well when it comes to ridding your body of different pollutants and toxins.

Chapter 4: Fruit Fasting

Fruit Fasting is considered to be one of the more popular types of fasting and it consists of ingesting only the freshest raw fruits. It is also a great fast for beginners as it is much easier on the body. It would also offer the individual a number of choices as to which fruit to use and much like the other fasting varieties, you can also create your own routine, one that fits well with your lifestyle and needs. This type of fasting, just like other methods, would create an environment in which your body can heal itself and rid itself of different toxins, and poisons-- excess fats included. This then results in us feeling much lighter and energetic, not to mention, fitter considering the fact that we have burned excess fat stores.

One Fruit Fast, is a kind of mono-diet where you would need to stick to one type of fruit for the duration of the fast itself. The most cleansing fruits would be grapes, citrus and apples. For first-timers, this is a great start. It would enable you to learn a lot about yourself and how much discomfort you would be able to tolerate. Usually, this lasts only a couple of days and not much preparation is really needed.

Any Fruit Fast, quite unlike the one fruit fast, this allows you to eat any fruit that you like as long as you stick to eating just fruits-- making sure that it is also of the raw variety. Apples, bananas, melons, grapes, citrus and mangoes would be great for this kind of fast as they are all known to be very detoxifying. While this is a popular diet for many, do note that there are certain fruit types that don't go well together such as those of an acidic nature and sweet ones. So do keep your combinations to a minimum and avoid eating citruses, and melons by themselves.

Fruit Fasting Tips:

1. Organic fruit is the preferred choice but it isn't always available. Instead, try to go for the highest quality fruits that you can find, especially for the ones in season.

2. Fruit fasting tends to be more comfortable to do in warmer climates or warmer months. For winter, rice fasting might be the better choice for you.

3. As much as you can, do avoid eating on the fly and make sure that you give enough attention to your daily meals. Just because it's small, it doesn't mean that you can give it less attention. Studies have shown that people tend to feel fuller if they focus more on the sensation of eating and remain conscious of it. So when you do sit down to eat, avoid doing other things that might distract you from it.

4. If you're doing a one fruit fast and using apple or citrus, do eat at least 1 to 2 fruits for every meal. 4 fruits for the whole day should be good enough to get you through what you need to get done.

So there you have it, a basic overview of fruit fasting as well as some tips on how you can get started. Remember, once you get the hang of things, you should be able to easily come up with a routine of your own that suits your needs and preferences well. You may also choose to consult a dietitian when it comes to this matter in order to make sure that you're not going overboard with it.

Chapter 5: Rice Fasting

It might seem like a strange notion but yes, you can certainly fast on rice. Fasting on brown rice, is, in fact, an ancient practice. It certainly is a milder form of fasting but serves the purpose well, offering the same benefits that all other methods can, including weight loss. Though, much like the others, it also has its own unique advantage. Among then, the alleviation of digestive troubles that you might be experiencing at the moment.

Even fasting for a few days can significantly help in decreasing the symptoms of your digestive troubles. Some of the problems targeted by it include allergies, diverticulitis, ulcers and irritable bowel syndrome. Some of these can be quite expensive to treat and would also require multiple visits to the doctor just for the symptoms to completely go away, luckily you don't have to go through that lengthy process. These can all be managed through a simple diet change. This is where the rice fasting enters the picture. Fasting for a few days would not only give your digestive system a rest, it would also re-balance it and alleviate acute symptoms.

Brown Rice Fasting: Gentler and smoother

This kind of fasting has the potential to be more stabilizing when compared to other varieties. Brown rice, as you may or may not know, is actually a complex carb which metabolizes and provides energy producing sugars gradually. When compared to fruit that is made up of simple sugars which are also quickly metabolized. This means that you wouldn't experience the same highs and lows that people go through when eating fruit, thus making it far more soothing and calming.

If you're going to be fasting cold weather or colder climates, then it would be far more comfortable if you do this with brown rice as it can actually be more warming when compared to other types of fasts. Water fasts can actually cause more discomfort because of its intensely detoxifying effect. While fasting on brown rice would still carry its own side effects, if you will, these would be much milder and also much easier to deal with.

Tips for fasting on brown rice:

1. Soak the grains to increase nutritional value. The thing with more modern methods of preparing rice is that it tends to be insufficient and in some cases, hinders the nutrients from full absorption. One of the newest studies also show that grains should be soaked and fermented before it gets cooked. This is a process that's very similar to soaking beans the night before cooking. In doing this, we're able to improve both benefits and nutritional value thus making it even better for fasting.

2. Plan on only taking 3 to 6 cups each day, moderation is key.

3. Do make sure that you only consume whole grain rice. Ayurveda also recommends that brown Basmati rice be used as this is the most balanced compared to the others. However, it isn't necessary and as long as you stick to something whole grain then it should be just as good.

4. Make sure that the rice itself is cooked properly and thoroughly. Why? This is because properly cooked rice

provides easier digestion as well as greater nutrient absorption.

5. Adding some sea salt to your rice is acceptable, especially if it's natural and of high quality. Salted sesame seeds are also a good addition for these are alkalizing and contains generous amounts of calcium. You may also choose to add a strip of seaweed to your rice or even a small amount of miso, it would deliver the same effect. Some cayenne pepper would also add warmth to it.

6. Adding a teaspoon of ghee or even butter would be fine as well. Saturated fats are actually essential if you want to achieve a healthier body overall. Butter contains a number of different essential vitamins. For strict vegans, a good alternative would be virgin coconut oil. These fats are actually known to help when it comes to getting rid of fat-soluble toxins and are needed when it comes to repairing damaged tissues.

7. Do resist the temptation to reheat your rice in a microwave and instead, steam it using a vegetable steamer or the stove top. This is the best way of doing things as you can avoid using too much heat and burning your rice. You can also just choose to eat it at room temperature of you are not too picky. It doesn't make any difference nor does it affect the nutritional value of the rice itself.

Rice fasting, as mentioned earlier, is great for colder climates and would also work well for beginners as it isn't as extreme as the other fasting diets but provides the same benefits, as well as a few other advantages. This could be great for individuals who do a lot on a daily basis and could use the energy that the rice would be able to provide them with. Again, do talk this over with your physician or dietitian as they would be able to advise you properly as to how you could get started with it.

Chapter 6: Fasting Tips

First time doing a fast? Well, let these tips steer you into the right direction and get you off nice and easy, without so much trouble. After all, you wouldn't want your first fasting diet to be traumatizing, right? So, let's get started.

1. Preparation. You can prepare for fasting by conditioning yourself to eat lighter and fewer meals for some days prior to actually doing the fast. The length of your preparation would be based upon the intensity and length of your planned fast. Do keep in mind that the longer or more intense your chosen fast is, the higher the number of days when it comes to preparing for it. If you drink caffeinated beverages on the regular, it would be helpful to slowly wean yourself off of it a few days prior as this would help you avoid any withdrawal headaches that might occur.

2. Keep yourself hydrated. Drink at least 2 quarts of water. Add a squeeze of lemon for a bit more flavor as well as much needed living enzymes. Remember to do this while you're fasting as it could also help ease any discomfort.

3. Ease up on your everyday activities. Opt for a lighter workload during your fast and remember never to overdo anything. Doing some moderate exercise should be fine in order to activate the body's fat burning but save your more strenuous duties for later, when you're past the fasting period. Doing yoga and some brisk walking are both well-suited to fasting so do give those a try.

4. Help your body when it comes to detoxification. Take the time to perform various breathing exercises as these would actually help you in shedding toxins as well as bring oxygen to your blood. Dry skin brushing is also known to improve the body's ability to detox by allow toxins to leave it through the skin as well as the lymphatic system.

5. Rest a lot. Allow yourself to take naps during the day or whenever you feel as if your energy is being depleted. Doing so would allow you to replenish the lost energy and when you wake up, you'll feel refreshed and re-energized.

Things to remember when breaking the fast:

Coming off of your fasting period does require a bit of extra attention and you cannot simply jump back into your old diet without any repercussion. It is important that you slowly ease your way back into it, in the same manner as you prepared for the fast. Doing it gradually would prevent shock to your body. Do keep in mind that much like preparing, the length as well as the intensity of your fast greatly affects and dictates how many days it might take for you to properly re-acclimate your body to eating regularly. Don't rush it, this is the important thing. Surely, you're already craving some of the meals you used to have but never rush it as you might end up damaging certain organs in the body if you do. Talk to your dietitian about this aspect of the diet, they would be able to advise you on what to do before and after your fast.

Just keep some of these tips in mind and make sure that you do this diet moderately for abuse of it can lead to various health consequences that are certainly not worth losing a few pounds for. Lose weight efficiently through fasting and do it the right way.

Conclusion

Thank you again for downloading this book!

I hope this book was able to help you to better understand how fasting works and the benefits that it can provide you with if done properly. There are many misrepresentations of this diet out there and most of the negativity lies in its abuse. Fasting is an effective way of losing weight and helping the body recover, one only needs to understand how to do it moderately.

The next step is to consider the options and if you're satisfied with what you've read, give the diet a try for yourself. Just remember to discuss your current condition with your physician so that they may ascertain if you're in the right health to undertake this diet.

Finally, if you enjoyed this book, please take the time to share your thoughts and post a review on Amazon. It'd be greatly appreciated!

Thank you and good luck!

www.ingramcontent.com/pod-product-compliance
Lightning Source LLC
Chambersburg PA
CBHW071328310526
45789CB00016B/1889